FACIAL CUPPING FOR BEGINNERS

Comprehensive Guide To Anti-Aging Techniques, Boosting Skin Health, And Enhancing Contour

DR SAWYER DIEGO

DISCLAMER

Nothing in this book should be interpreted as medical advice; it is meant exclusively for educational reasons. Regarding their specific health issues and treatment options, readers are urged to speak with licensed healthcare professionals. The publisher and author disclaim all liability for any errors or omissions in the material provided, as well as for any negative effects that may arise from using or abusing the information. Although every attempt has been taken to guarantee that the material in this book is correct as of the date of publishing, new research may have superseded some of the content because medical knowledge is always changing. It is recommended that readers confirm the most recent medical recommendations and guidelines. The reader of this book undertakes to release the author and publisher from any claims or liabilities resulting from the use of this information, and understands and accepts the inherent risks connected with healthcare decisions.

TABLE OF CONTENTS

ABOUT THE BOOK

"Facial Cupping for Beginners" is a crucial resource for anyone interested in learning more about the restorative powers of facial cupping therapy. It explores the history and origins of facial cupping, following its development from traditional practices to its current uses in skincare.

It also highlights the differences between facial and body cupping, with a focus on the specialized techniques and tools designed for sensitive facial skin.

Comprehending the science-backed advantages of facial cupping for skin health is crucial. Through improved circulation and lymphatic drainage, facial cupping reduces puffiness, improves the appearance of a youthful complexion, and facilitates the absorption of skincare products. When done properly, this therapy is safe and provides a comprehensive skincare regimen that can be easily incorporated into everyday routines.

The book starts with a thorough introduction to facial cupping for beginners, going over its mechanisms and safety measures. It then walks readers through the necessary equipment, such as various kinds of cupping tools and appropriate materials for facial treatments. The book also includes helpful advice on skin preparation, hygiene, and choosing oils or serums, emphasizing the significance of creating a workspace that is conducive to both safe and successful cupping sessions.

Advanced techniques, like combining cupping with Gua Sha or addressing specific skin concerns like acne or aging, offer versatility in treatment approaches. The fundamentals of facial cupping are thoroughly explained, from step-by-step procedures to varying methods like static and gliding cupping. Readers will learn about adjusting pressure and duration according to target areas on the face, along with common mistakes to avoid for optimal results.

The book also addresses common concerns about facial cupping, such as its safety, potential marks, and suitability for different skin types. Aftercare and maintenance are stressed to ensure the longevity and efficacy of facial cupping sessions. This includes developing a post-cupping skincare routine, properly cleaning and sterilizing tools, and monitoring skin reactions to adjust techniques as needed.

Comprehensive FAQs shed light on things like how often to have sessions, what to expect afterward, and how cupping therapy works to treat wrinkles and puffiness in the face. It also looks at new developments in facial cupping, like sustainability initiatives and cutting-edge techniques, giving an overview of how skincare therapies are developing.

Since facial cupping is becoming more and more popular due to its all-natural, non-invasive benefits, this book provide beginners with the information and self-assurance they need to start their journey towards healthier, more radiant skin.

CHAPTER ONE
FACIAL CUPPING OVERVIEW
DEFINITION OF FACIAL CUPPING

Face cupping is a non-invasive therapy that uses small suction cups to create a gentle vacuum on the skin's surface. It is thought to have originated from Chinese and Middle Eastern medicine practices that aimed to improve skin health and overall well-being thousands of years ago. In contrast to body cupping, which frequently leaves circular marks due to stronger suction, facial cupping uses softer suction to stimulate circulation, promote lymphatic drainage, and enhance collagen production.

The purpose of facial cupping is to massage the skin and underlying tissues by gently gliding or moving the cups in circular motions. The cups are usually made of glass or silicone to ensure a smooth glide over the skin. This helps to release tension, reduce puffiness, and encourage nutrient-rich blood flow to the skin's surface, promoting a radiant and youthful complexion. Facial cupping is often combined with facial oils or serums to enhance the gliding motion of the cups and nourish the skin.

Facial cupping is safe when done correctly and can be incorporated into skincare routines to address concerns like fine lines, wrinkles, dullness, and uneven skin tone. Frequent practice of facial cupping may also improve the absorption of skincare products, making it a versatile addition to both professional treatments and home skincare rituals. Beginners should understand the pressure needed to create suction without causing discomfort or bruising.

ADVANTAGES OF CUPPING YOUR FACE

Facial cupping is a popular option for people looking for natural skin care solutions because it has several advantages for skin health and appearance. Firstly, it can help reduce puffiness and promote a more defined facial contour by stimulating lymphatic drainage and circulation. Secondly, by improving blood flow to the skin's surface, facial cupping can also improve the delivery of oxygen and nutrients, which can lead to a complexion that is brighter and more rejuvenated.

Furthermore, regular facial cupping sessions can help to counteract these effects by promoting collagen synthesis, which over time will result in smoother and suppler skin. Collagen is a key protein responsible for skin elasticity and firmness, and as we age, our natural production of collagen declines, causing sagging skin and wrinkles.

Facial cupping also has the potential to help reduce the appearance of fine lines brought on by stress and repetitive facial expressions by relaxing facial muscles and releasing tension held in the jaw and face.

The gentle suction of the cups also promotes the detoxification of skin tissues by drawing impurities to the surface, which can further clarify the complexion and support overall skin health.

THE MECHANISM OF FACIAL CUPPING

To achieve different therapeutic effects, facial cupping typically involves applying the cups to different points on the face and moving them in specific patterns. This creates a gentle suction on the skin's surface, which helps to lift and massage the underlying tissues. Additionally, this suction stimulates circulation, promoting the flow of nutrient-rich blood to the skin cells and encouraging cellular repair and regeneration.

By improving lymphatic drainage in the face, facial cupping can reduce puffiness and congestion, resulting in a clearer and more radiant complexion. The gentle pulling action of the cups also encourages the release of fascia, the connective tissue that supports and separates muscles and organs. The suction effect of facial cupping also helps to stimulate the lymphatic system, which is crucial in removing toxins and waste products from the body.

Depending on the desired intensity and treatment area, different cup sizes and materials can be used for facial cupping. Glass cups offer a smoother glide over the skin, but silicone cups are more flexible and user-friendly. A lubricant, such as facial oil or serum, is necessary to help the cups move and avoid causing too much friction on the skin.

SAFETY AND PRECAUTIONS

Although most people find facial cupping to be safe, there are a few things to know to make sure you have a good and efficient experience. First and foremost, novices should start with a light suction and work their way up to a stronger suction as they gain more familiarity with the technique. This will help to avoid bruising or discomfort, especially on delicate areas of the face.

Facial cups should never be applied to broken or irritated skin because they can worsen inflammation and even lead to infection. People who have rosacea or active acne should also see a skincare specialist before beginning any facial cupping regimen to prevent making their conditions worse.

It's normal to experience mild redness or slight bruising after a facial cupping session, especially if the cups were used with stronger suction; this usually goes away in a few days. You can help relieve any temporary discomfort and speed up the healing process of your skin by applying a soothing moisturizer or cooling gel.

Finally, it's important to remember that using facial cups requires good hygiene. To avoid bacterial buildup and to ensure hygienic conditions for your skincare routine, thoroughly clean the cups before and after each use.

With consistent use and adherence to safety precautions, facial cupping can be a helpful addition to your skincare routine, promoting healthier, more radiant skin over time.

STARTING: REQUIRED EQUIPMENT

First, choose high-quality facial cups made of silicone or glass, preferably with a variety of sizes to accommodate different areas of the face. Because silicone cups are flexible and easy to handle, they are often recommended for beginners. These are the essential tools needed to start facial cupping at home and ensure a safe and effective experience.

Next, select an appropriate face oil or serum to lubricate the cups as they glide over the skin. Look for non-comedogenic, lightweight products that work well for your skin type to improve the gliding action of the cups while also providing skin nourishment.

Apply a thin layer of facial oil or serum to the treatment area after gently patting your skin dry with a soft towel. This helps to create a barrier between the cups and your skin, minimizing friction and potential discomfort during the session. Before beginning, thoroughly cleanse your face to remove makeup, dirt, and excess oil.

Start with light suction and work your way outward in gentle upward strokes from the center of your face; use smaller cups on sensitive areas like the lips and eye area, and adjust the suction strength to your comfort level; don't stay in one spot for too long to avoid bruises and to guarantee even circulation throughout your face.

Following a facial cupping session, resume your usual skincare regimen (moisturize, apply sunscreen if you want to go outside), and thoroughly wash the cups with warm water and mild soap. Let the cups air dry before storing them in a dry, clean area for later use.

Through increased circulation and lymphatic drainage, facial cupping can promote a brighter, more youthful complexion. With regular practice and attention to technique, it can become a calming and useful addition to your skincare routine.

CHAPTER TWO
COMPREHENDING FACE CUPPING
HISTORY AND ORIGINS

Originating thousands of years ago, cupping therapy was thought to balance the body's yin and yang energies by creating suction on the skin's surface. Over time, this practice evolved into various forms, including facial cupping, which specifically targets the delicate skin of the face and neck. Originally, facial cupping was used as a method to stimulate acupuncture points and improve circulation.

While its traditional roots are in Chinese medicine, modern practitioners have modified the technique to suit contemporary beauty and wellness practices.

By understanding its historical context, practitioners and users alike can appreciate how facial cupping has transcended cultural boundaries to become a widely recognized skincare therapy. In modern times, facial cupping has gained popularity as a non-invasive cosmetic treatment aimed at rejuvenating the skin and reducing the signs of aging.

CONTEMPORARY USES

Today, practitioners use specially designed silicone or glass cups to create a gentle suction on the skin's surface, which lifts the facial tissues and stimulates blood flow and lymphatic drainage, which can reduce puffiness and promote a more radiant complexion. Facial cupping's modern applications go beyond traditional Chinese medicine to encompass a range of therapeutic and cosmetic benefits.

Modern facial cupping techniques emphasize safety, comfort, and customizable treatment options tailored to individual skin types and concerns. Besides its cosmetic benefits, these techniques often incorporate essential oils or serums to maximize the effectiveness of the treatment. These products are applied to the face before cupping, allowing the cups to glide smoothly and providing additional nourishment to the skin.

DISTINCTIONS FROM BODY CUPPING

The technique and goal of facial cupping are very different from those of traditional body cupping techniques: body cupping targets muscle tension and pain relief by using larger cups and stronger suction; facial cupping uses smaller, softer cups to gently lift the skin; the suction created in facial cupping is much milder and is intended to stimulate the superficial layers of the skin without leaving marks or bruising.

Furthermore, while body cupping may involve more intense suction to address deeper muscular issues and promote relaxation, facial cupping focuses primarily on improving skin elasticity, reducing fine lines and wrinkles, and improving overall skin health and appearance. Practitioners and users need to recognize these differences to ensure the safe and effective application of cupping therapy according to specific treatment goals.

ADVANTAGES FOR SKIN HEALTH

Facial cupping is a popular option for people looking for natural, non-invasive skincare treatments because it has many benefits for skin health. It reduces puffiness and promotes a brighter, younger-looking complexion by stimulating blood circulation and lymphatic drainage. Over time, the gentle suction of the cups can improve skin tone and firmness by encouraging the production of collagen.

Regular treatments may also enhance the penetration and effectiveness of skincare products, allowing for better absorption of nutrients and moisture into the skin. As a result, facial cupping is often recommended for people looking to maintain healthier-looking skin without invasive procedures or harsh chemicals. Additionally, by promoting cell regeneration and tissue repair, facial cupping can help diminish the appearance of fine lines, wrinkles, and scars.

SCIENTIFIC SUPPORT

Studies have demonstrated that facial cupping can increase blood circulation and lymphatic drainage, which are crucial for detoxifying the skin and reducing fluid buildup that contributes to puffiness. The mechanical action of cupping also stimulates fibroblast cells to produce collagen and elastin, which are essential proteins for skin structure and elasticity. A growing body of scientific research is confirming the benefits of facial cupping and validating its usefulness in skincare and wellness practices.

In addition, studies have shown that facial cupping can improve skin tone and texture, as well as lessen the appearance of wrinkles and fine lines. These results corroborate anecdotal reports from practitioners and clients who report smoother, more radiant skin following regular cupping treatments.

CHAPTER THREE
DIFFERENT CUPPING TOOL TYPES
VARIOUS CUPPING TOOLS

Unlike traditional body cupping, facial cupping uses specialized instruments made for smaller, more delicate areas of the face. The most common instruments used are silicone cups, glass cups, and plastic cups. Silicone cups are popular because they are flexible, easy to use, gentle on the skin, and allow for better control over suction intensity. Glass cups are another option because they are durable and effective at creating suction; they provide a stronger suction than silicone cups but need to be handled carefully to avoid breaking. Plastic cups, on the other hand, are lightweight and less likely to break than glass cups, making them suitable for beginners.

While glass cups are more fragile, they have a stronger suction that can effectively lift and tone the skin; plastic cups strike a balance between durability and effectiveness, making them a practical choice for those new to facial cupping; silicone cups are ideal for beginners due to their ease of use and gentle application; they are often recommended for facial cupping as they can be easily manipulated to target specific areas like around the eyes or lips.

SELECTING THE APPROPRIATE SIZE

For successful facial cupping, it is important to choose the right size cup. There are several cup sizes, from small to large, and each has a different function on the face. Smaller cups are generally better for beginners because they are easier to handle and fit on facial contours like the lips, nose, and eyes. Larger cups are better for broader areas like the forehead and cheeks, but they may be more difficult to use without hurting.

Try experimenting with different sizes to find the cup size that works best for your unique facial contours and skincare goals. Smaller cups are ideal for targeting fine lines, wrinkles, and puffiness around delicate areas.

They provide precise suction without overwhelming the skin. Larger cups are suitable for covering larger areas, promoting circulation and lymphatic drainage across the face.

MATERIALS EMPLOYED

The materials used to make facial cupping instruments have a big impact on how safe and effective they are. Medical-grade silicone, which is flexible and hypoallergenic, is typically used to make silicone cups. This material guarantees a mild but strong suction that won't irritate or damage the skin. Glass cups are made of heat-resistant, long-lasting glass that can withstand repeated use and sterilization. This glass provides a strong suction that lifts and firms the skin, improving circulation and collagen production. Plastic cups are typically made of lightweight, BPA-free plastic that is durable and easy to handle during facial cupping sessions.

Plastic cups offer a balance between durability and effectiveness, suitable for beginners looking to explore facial cupping without committing to more delicate materials. Glass cups provide a stronger suction for deeper tissue manipulation and are favored for their durability and long-term use. Silicone cups are popular for their user-friendly design and gentle application, making them ideal for beginners and those with sensitive skin.

COMPARING DIFFERENT SUCTION TECHNIQUES

To achieve the desired skin care results, facial cupping uses two different suction techniques: dynamic cupping, which involves moving cups across the face in gentle gliding motions to stimulate lymphatic drainage and enhance absorption of skincare products, and static cupping, which involves placing cups on specific areas of the face without moving and allowing suction to draw the skin upwards, effectively promoting circulation and reducing puffiness.

The decision between static and dynamic cupping techniques comes down to personal preferences and skincare goals. Static cupping is easy to use and perfect for novices looking for a basic yet effective facial rejuvenation procedure. It offers instant lifting effects and encourages the production of natural collagen. Dynamic cupping, on the other hand, is more massage-like, improving blood flow and enhancing the delivery of nutrients to the skin. It can be customized to target specific issues like under-eye bags or jawline definition.

ACCESSORIES REQUIRED

A facial cleanser is advised before each session to ensure the skin is clean and free of makeup or impurities, maximizing the benefits of facial cupping. Cotton pads or tissues can be used to remove excess oil or serum after each session, leaving the skin refreshed and hydrated. Facial oils or serums are essential for lubricating the skin and creating a barrier between the cup and the face.

This allows cups to glide smoothly without pulling or tugging on delicate skin.

A timer or stopwatch helps track session duration, ensuring consistent treatment times for optimal results. Storage pouches or containers keep cups organized and protected when not in use, prolonging their lifespan. These accessories complement the facial cupping experience, making it easier for beginners to incorporate into their skincare routine successfully and comfortably. A mirror is also helpful for beginners to monitor cup placement and ensure even coverage across the face.

CHAPTER FOUR

HOW TO GET READY FOR FACE CUPPING

TIPS FOR SKIN PREPARATION

It's important to properly prepare your skin before starting a facial cupping procedure. To start, make sure your face is clean and free of residues that could interfere with the cupping process by using a gentle cleanser that is appropriate for your skin type. After cleansing, pat dry with a fresh towel.

Applying a facial oil or serum next will help the cups glide more smoothly over your skin. Look for an oil that is safe to use on your face, preferably non-comedogenic to prevent clogged pores, and gently massage it into the areas of your face where you intend to use the cups.

Before beginning the cupping procedure, make sure your skin is hydrated and plump. You may also want to think about using an exfoliant or facial scrub to help remove dead skin cells and encourage better circulation. This step can enhance the effectiveness of the cupping treatment by allowing the cups to create a stronger suction on the skin.

HYGIENE PRACTICES

To avoid infections or skin irritations, it's important to practice good hygiene when doing facial cupping. To start, wash your hands well with soap and water before handling the cups or touching your face. This will lessen the chance that dirt or bacteria will get onto your skin while the treatment is being performed.

Before using any cup, make sure it is clean and sanitized. You can wash it with warm water and a small amount of detergent, then rinse it well and let it air dry. If the cup is broken or has sharp edges, don't use it to avoid cutting your skin.

Disposable cups should be thrown away after every treatment to uphold hygienic standards.

By adhering to these guidelines, you can guarantee a secure and efficient face-cupping experience without endangering the health of your skin. Reusable cups should be kept in a clean, dry place between usages.

CHOOSING THE RIGHT OILS OR SERUMS

Choosing the right oils or serums for facial cupping can increase the benefits of the treatment. Look for lightweight oils that absorb quickly into the skin, like argan oil, jojoba oil, or rosehip seed oil. These oils are great for cupping and facial massage because they nourish and hydrate the skin without leaving a greasy afterglow.

As an alternative, you can choose serums designed to address particular skin concerns, such as those that increase skin elasticity or fight aging. To reduce the chance of allergic reactions or skin irritation, look for products free of harsh chemicals and synthetic smells.

Apply a few drops of the oil or serum evenly over your face and gently massage it in until absorbed, preparing your skin for the cupping process and maximizing the overall benefits of the treatment. Before applying the oil or serum, do a patch test on a small area of your skin to ensure you don't have any negative reactions.

SETTING UP YOUR WORKSPACE

A well-organized and cozy workspace is crucial to a successful facial cupping session. To begin, choose a peaceful, well-lit spot where you can unwind while receiving the treatment, and make sure you have a spotless surface on which to set your cups, oils, and other necessary tools.

Methodically organize your equipment to prevent confusion or interruptions throughout the treatment. Keep a fresh towel or tissue close by to remove any extra oil or perspiration that may build up.

To help you relax and get the most out of your facial cupping experience, try playing relaxing music or utilizing aromatherapy to create a quiet ambiance.

By carefully organizing your workstation, you may have a more pleasant and productive treatment session.

SAFETY CONSIDERATIONS

Just like any skincare treatment, facial cupping involves taking precautions to minimize risks or discomfort. To start, make sure the cups you use are made of safe materials, like silicone, or are specifically designed for use on the face. Avoid using cups that are too rigid or have sharp edges, as these can damage skin.

Always move the cups in upward motions to facilitate lymphatic drainage and blood circulation without pulling or stretching the skin unduly. When applying the cups, use mild suction and avoid putting them in one spot for too long to prevent bruising or redness.

Use a calming moisturizer or face lotion to nourish the skin and minimize redness or sensitivity after the treatment.

If you continue to feel uncomfortable or irritated, stop using facial cupping and see a skincare specialist.

You may reap the benefits of face cupping while preserving the integrity and health of your skin by putting safety first and adhering to these recommendations.

CHAPTER FIVE

FUNDAMENTAL METHODS OF FACE CUPPING

METHODICAL PROCESS

To ensure smooth gliding of the cups, cleanse your face thoroughly and apply a facial oil or serum. Start with a small cup to become familiar with the technique. Place the cup on the desired area of the face, usually starting from the forehead or cheeks. Squeeze the cup gently to create suction. Glide the cup across the skin using upward or circular motions, avoiding sensitive areas like the eyes and lips. Repeat this process for each section of the face, maintaining gentle pressure to avoid bruising.

Frequent use of facial cupping can help improve skin tone, reduce puffiness, and enhance the overall radiance of your complexion. As you become more accustomed to the procedure, you can modify the suction strength and duration based on the sensitivity and tolerance of your skin. After the session, hydrate the skin and minimize any temporary redness.

VARIOUS CUPPING TECHNIQUES (GLIDING VS. STATIC)

There are two main techniques used in facial cupping: gliding and static. Static cupping is where the cups are placed on certain points of the face and left there for a few seconds to several minutes. It is useful for targeting acupressure points and encouraging relaxation. Gliding cupping, on the other hand, is where the cups are moved continuously across the skin to help stimulate circulation more dynamically. It can also help reduce fine lines and promote lymphatic drainage.

For gliding cupping, use a facial oil or serum to facilitate smooth movement of the cups and prevent pulling on the skin. Maintain a consistent pressure and avoid excessive suction that may cause bruising or irritation. Both methods can be combined within a single session to maximize the benefits of facial cupping. When practicing static cupping, make sure the cups are securely suctioned to the skin without causing discomfort. Start with shorter durations and gradually increase the time as your skin adapts to the treatment.

GUIDELINES FOR PRESSURE AND DURATION

Depending on your skin sensitivity and treatment objectives, you should modify the pressure and length of your facial cupping sessions. Start with light to moderate pressure and gradually increase the suction as your skin adjusts to the cups; avoid applying too much pressure as this can result in bruises or broken capillaries. Start with shorter sessions, usually lasting 5 to 10 minutes, and extend them as you gain experience and see how your skin reacts.

Smaller cups and lighter suction are recommended for sensitive areas like the mouth and around the eyes. If you notice any redness or irritation on your skin, adjust the pressure accordingly.

Facial cupping should be soothing and comfortable, encouraging a gentle pulling sensation rather than pain. Use a calming moisturizer or facial serum after each session to nourish your skin and aid in its recovery.

TARGET FACE AREAS

Applying facial cupping to different parts of the face can help target particular issues and improve overall skin health. Common target areas include the neck, jawline, forehead, and cheeks. Start by concentrating on one area at a time, working your way outward from the center of the face, using smaller cups for more delicate areas like the under-eye area and larger cups for more expansive areas like the forehead or cheeks.

Always move the cups in upward motions to counteract gravity and promote a lifting effect. Tailor the treatment to your specific concerns, whether it's minimizing fine lines, improving overall radiance, or reducing puffiness.

For the forehead, use upward strokes to help lift the brows and smooth out wrinkles. For the cheeks, use circular motions to enhance circulation and improve skin tone. For the jawline, use gentle gliding motions to reduce tension and define the contours of the face.

TYPICAL ERRORS TO STEER CLEAR OF

Avoiding common mistakes that can compromise the safety and efficacy of facial cupping treatments is crucial. For example, using cups with excessive suction can result in bruising, broken capillaries, or discomfort. Instead, start with a gentle suction and increase it gradually, paying close attention to how your skin reacts.

Another common error is not applying a facial oil or serum before cupping. This can result in pulling and friction on the skin, which can cause redness or irritation. A small coating of oil should be applied to maintain the skin barrier and enable the cups to glide smoothly.

Move the cups often to minimize static suction marks and to uniformly distribute the advantages of facial cupping across the face; avoid leaving them in one spot for extended periods, especially on delicate areas like the cheeks or around the eyes.

Remember to take proper care of your skin after facial cupping. Use a calming serum or moisturizer to hydrate the skin and lessen any transient redness. Clean the cups regularly with mild soap and water to maintain hygiene and prevent bacterial buildup. By avoiding these common blunders and using facial cupping correctly, you can reap the benefits of facial cupping and encourage healthier, more radiant skin.

CHAPTER SIX
ADVANCED METHODS FOR CUPPING THE FACE
COMBINING ONE THERAPY WITH ANOTHER (GUA SHA, FOR EXAMPLE)

Together, these therapies enhance their benefits and provide a holistic approach to skincare. Gua Sha, which involves scraping the skin with a tool to improve circulation and lymphatic drainage, complements facial cupping by further stimulating blood flow and promoting detoxification. Facial cupping and other therapeutic techniques like Gua Sha can be combined effectively to enhance overall facial rejuvenation.

To combine facial cupping with Gua Sha, first, ensure that your skin is clean and moisturized, and apply a facial oil to help the tools glide smoothly. Next, use Gua Sha to gently scrape the contours of your face, encouraging lymphatic drainage and decreasing puffiness.

Finally, use silicone cups for facial cupping, which will lift and tone your facial muscles, increasing circulation and stimulating the production of collagen. This combination therapy will not only improve the elasticity of your skin but also help reduce fine lines and promote a radiant complexion.

This combination therapy is a great complement to any skincare regimen looking for natural rejuvenation techniques because regular use can result in noticeable improvements in skin tone and texture.

BOOSTING OUTCOMES WITH ESSENTIAL OILS

By adding therapeutic benefits and targeting particular skin concerns, essential oils can greatly improve the results of facial cupping.

When choosing essential oils for facial cupping, take into account their anti-inflammatory, antioxidant, and antimicrobial effects, which can effectively address a variety of skin issues.

To use essential oils in facial cupping, dilute a few drops of your preferred oil in a carrier oil that is appropriate for applying to the face. Apply this mixture to the skin before using the cups, making sure to distribute it evenly for optimal absorption and benefit. As the cups lift and sculpt the face, the oils deeply penetrate the skin layers, nourishing and hydrating as they do so.

Choosing your essential oil blend according to skin type and concerns allows for a customized skincare experience that maximizes the benefits of facial cupping, promoting overall skin health and radiance. Popular essential oils for facial cupping include lavender for calming sensitive skin, tea tree for acne-prone skin, and rosehip seed oil for anti-aging benefits.

HANDLING PARTICULAR SKIN ISSUES (E.G., AGING, ACNE)

With targeted solutions available for common skin concerns like acne and signs of aging, facial cupping is a versatile therapy for improving the health and appearance of skin. In the case of acne-prone skin, lymphatic drainage stimulation and inflammation reduction help to clear congestion, and gentle suction helps to remove excess oil and toxins, minimizing breakouts and gradually promoting clearer skin.

To treat indications of aging, facial cupping lifts, and tones facial muscles, which in turn restores firmness and elasticity to the skin, giving the appearance of young skin. It also promotes collagen synthesis and enhances blood circulation, which helps to decrease fine lines, wrinkles, and drooping.

Applying facial cupping consistently to address individual skin needs can result in noticeable improvements in complexion and texture, promoting overall skin rejuvenation. Targeted techniques, such as focusing on problematic areas with slower, more deliberate movements, can help achieve effective results. Suction intensity can be adjusted based on skin sensitivity and desired outcomes, ensuring a comfortable and effective treatment.

USING FACIAL CUPPING TO UNWIND

Facial cupping is a popular cosmetic procedure that also has a calming impact on the muscles in the face and enhances overall well-being. It is a great way to add relaxation to self-care routines since it releases tension and stress stored in the facial muscles.

To benefit from the calming effects of facial cupping, set up a peaceful space with soft lighting and relaxing music. First, apply a facial oil to improve glide and comfort. Then, using a light suction, move the cups slowly and rhythmically along the contours of the face, concentrating on tense areas like the forehead, temples, and jawline.

Adding facial cupping to regular skincare routines not only improves skin health but also fosters overall relaxation and stress relief, supporting holistic well-being. This technique releases facial muscle tightness and promotes blood flow and lymphatic drainage, stimulating a sense of rejuvenation and relaxation.

ADDING CUPPING TO SKINCARE PRACTICES

The effectiveness and sustainability of face cupping as a holistic skincare technique are increased when it is incorporated into daily skincare routines. Over time, regular cupping can help you retain skin elasticity, encourage lymphatic drainage, and improve the overall tone and texture of your skin.

When incorporating facial cupping into your skincare routine, start with a clean face and use a facial oil or serum to ensure that the cups glide smoothly. Next, lightly suction the skin and move the cups upward and outward across the face, focusing on various areas like the forehead, jawline, and cheeks. You can adjust the suction intensity based on your comfort level and skin sensitivity.

Consistently using facial cupping as part of your daily skincare routine allows for consistent and noticeable improvements in skin health, making it a beneficial practice for long-term beauty and wellness.

Regular use of facial cupping reduces the appearance of fine lines and wrinkles, enhances the absorption of skincare products, and helps to detoxify the skin by promoting circulation and lymphatic drainage, resulting in a brighter and more youthful complexion.

CHAPTER SEVEN
MAINTENANCE AND AFTERCARE
AFTER-CUPPING SKINCARE PROTOCOL

Following up with a proper skincare routine is essential to maximizing the benefits of a facial cupping session and ensuring that your skin stays healthy and radiant. Begin by gently cleansing your face with a mild cleanser to remove any residue from the cupping oils and encourage circulation. Pat dry with a soft towel to avoid needless friction. Next, replenish moisture and nourish your skin with a hydrating serum or facial oil. This step is crucial because cupping can temporarily increase blood flow, which makes your skin more receptive to nutrients.

After the serum, use a skin-type-appropriate moisturizer to seal in moisture and shield your skin barrier; stay away from heavy creams that can clog pores; if you're cupping at night, use a night cream or mask to encourage overnight rejuvenation; and if you're staying indoors, wear sunscreen in the morning to prevent UV damage. This routine will guarantee that your skin is balanced and radiant after every cupping session, promoting long-term benefits.

INSTRUMENT SANITIZATION AND STERILIZATION

To prevent bacteria and ensure safe and effective facial cupping sessions, it is imperative to keep cupping tools sterile and clean. To start, wash the cups thoroughly with warm water and mild soap after each use. Use a soft brush or cloth to remove any oils or residues that may have accumulated during the session. Rinse the cups well to make sure there is no soap residue left that could irritate the skin when you use them again.

To ensure that the cups are safe for reuse after washing, sterilize them using a suitable method, such as boiling water or alcohol wipes; alternatively, wipe the cups with alcohol and let them air dry before storing them in a clean, dry place. To ensure that hygiene standards are maintained, make sure to sterilize not only the cups but also any accessories, like suction pumps or applicators.

You can safely and effectively reap the benefits of facial cupping by incorporating proper cleaning and sterilization into your routine, which not only prolongs the life of your cupping tools but also shields your skin from potential infections or negative reactions. Regularly inspect your cups for signs of wear or damage, such as cracks or discoloration, which may indicate the need for replacement.

REGULARITY OF SESSIONS

The number of facial cupping sessions that you should schedule depends on your specific skin type and goals. If you're new to the process, it's best to schedule one session per week to give your skin time to adjust and see any reactions. As you gain confidence in the technique and your skin's response, you can progressively schedule two or three sessions per week, depending on your skin's tolerance and desired outcomes.

Following each session, pay close attention to your skin's reaction; some people may experience mild redness or slight bruising, which is normal and usually goes away in a few days; if you notice prolonged redness, irritation, or discomfort, cut down on the number of sessions or seek advice from a skincare professional; consistency is key to getting the best results from facial cupping, so figure out a routine that suits your needs and lifestyle.

One way to reap the benefits of facial cupping safely and effectively is to adjust the frequency based on your skin's response and maintain a balanced approach. Another way to avoid potential sensitivity or adverse reactions is to allow your skin time to rest in between sessions. Finally, if you use other skincare treatments or products in your routine, think about how they interact with facial cupping.

OBSERVING SKIN RESPONSES

To guarantee safety and efficacy, it is imperative to observe how your skin reacts both during and after facial cupping sessions. During the session, note how your skin reacts to the suction and movement of the cups; mild redness or temporary marks where the cups were applied are normal and indicate increased circulation and oxygen flow to the skin.

Following the treatment, keep an eye out for any persistent redness, irritation, or unusual sensitivity on your skin.

These could indicate overstimulation or a negative reaction to the technique. If you experience chronic pain or see changes in the texture or tone of your skin, stop cupping temporarily and seek advice from a skincare specialist.

You can reap the benefits of facial cupping while lowering the possibility of potential side effects by monitoring the state of your skin in between sessions, looking for any trends or concerns that may surface, and adjusting your cupping technique or frequency accordingly to keep your skin healthy and responsive.

TECHNIQUES TO MODIFY FOR SENSITIVITY

You can modify facial cupping techniques to suit varying degrees of sensitivity and to make sure that beginners have a comfortable experience. To minimize the risk of bruising or discomfort, try using shorter sessions with lighter suction pressure. This will still encourage lymphatic drainage and circulation.

Try experimenting with different cup sizes and techniques to find what works best for you without putting undue pressure or irritation on your skin. Silicone cups are often gentler on the skin compared to traditional glass or plastic cups, making them ideal for beginners or individuals with sensitive skin.

During and after each session, observe how your skin reacts; if you feel uncomfortable or have persistent redness, lower the suction intensity or shorten the cupping session. Take pauses in between sessions to give your skin time to repair and regenerate; if your skin responds well to the technique, gradually increase the suction intensity or duration.

You can reap the therapeutic benefits of facial cupping while reducing the risk of negative reactions by customizing your cupping techniques based on your skin's sensitivity and feedback. Patience and consistency are essential for achieving the best possible results, so be sure to customize your approach to make sure you have a safe and enjoyable experience.

CHAPTER EIGHT

TYPICAL FEARS REGARDING FACIAL CUPPING

IS IT SAFE TO CUP YOUR FACE?

The safety of facial cupping, a traditional therapy that is becoming more and more popular in modern skincare routines, is a concern for novices. When done properly, facial cupping is generally safe and non-invasive, providing several benefits like improved circulation, decreased puffiness, and enhanced skin elasticity.

To prevent any negative effects, it is important to use the proper size and type of cups suitable for delicate facial skin. To avoid misusing the technique, novices should make sure they fully understand it or seek guidance from a qualified practitioner.

To safely perform facial cupping, you should first cleanse your skin and apply light massage oil to facilitate the smooth glide of the small silicone cups.

This technique helps promote a natural glow and reduce the appearance of fine lines by stimulating blood flow and lymphatic drainage. It's important to keep in mind that excessive suction or leaving the cups in one place for an extended period can result in bruising or broken capillaries, so proceed with caution and always prioritize your skin's sensitivity and tolerance levels.

Beginners should prioritize safety by utilizing the right techniques and materials, even if face cupping may be a helpful addition to skincare routines. Start with tiny cups, maintain mild suction, and refrain from overdoing it to enjoy the rejuvenating effects without compromising skin health.

DOES CUPPING CAUSE TRACES?

Beginners who are interested in facial cupping frequently wonder if it will leave visible marks on their skin. When done properly, however, facial cupping usually leaves little to no marks; the secret is to use light suction and move the cups frequently to avoid stagnant blood pooling, which causes discoloration. Body cupping, on the other hand, frequently leaves circular bruises due to stronger suction and longer application times.

To reduce the chance of scarring, novices should work slowly when performing facial cupping techniques and stay out of one spot for longer. Silicone cups made especially for the face are a good choice because they have enough suction without pressing too hard on the skin. You should also use a small amount of oil or serum to make the cups move more easily and to lessen friction, which will improve the whole experience and lessen the possibility of skin irritation.

While temporary marks or slight pinkness may result from increased blood circulation during facial cupping, these effects are usually mild and disappear quickly; beginners can still benefit from facial cupping without having to worry too much about visible marks on their skin as long as they use the right techniques and tools.

CAN ANYBODY PERFORM FACE CUPPING?

Most people can benefit from facial cupping, but some conditions may need to be treated with caution or after consulting a healthcare provider. For example, people with rosacea, sensitive skin, or active acne should proceed with caution when using facial cupping to prevent aggravating these conditions. Pregnant women, people with open wounds or skin infections, and people with sensitive skin should also avoid using facial cupping until they have spoken with their healthcare provider.

To maximize the overall effectiveness of facial cupping, use silicone cups made especially for the purpose, starting with a gentle suction level to see how your skin reacts.

The technique should be performed in a well-lit area on clean, moisturized skin to allow for smooth cup movement. Excessive suction or long cupping sessions should be avoided to minimize the risk of skin irritation or discomfort.

Most people can safely undergo facial cupping, but before beginning, beginners should think about their skin type and any pre-existing skin conditions. Personalized guidance can be obtained by speaking with a healthcare provider or skincare expert, ensuring a successful and enjoyable facial cupping experience.

LONG-TERM ADVANTAGES OVER SHORT-TERM CONSEQUENCES

A common question among novices investigating facial cupping is how to strike a balance between the immediate results—which can include a radiant glow and improved facial contouring—and the longer-term benefits. The immediate effects of facial cupping usually include immediate skin plumping, reduced puffiness, and enhanced circulation due to the temporary suction effect.

Consistency is key to achieving long-term results, as facial cupping becomes a part of a comprehensive skincare routine.

Regular facial cupping sessions can contribute to improved skin elasticity, reduced fine lines, and enhanced lymphatic drainage over time. The gentle suction encourages collagen production and stimulates circulation, promoting a healthier complexion with continued use.

Beginners should gradually increase the frequency of facial cupping sessions as their skin adjusts to the treatment, starting with short sessions to maximize both the short-term and long-term benefits. By keeping a balanced approach and emphasizing proper technique, beginners can enjoy both immediate and long-lasting improvements in skin health and appearance.

Facial cupping provides instant benefits like decreased puffiness and increased circulation, but regular use also improves skin elasticity and reduces fine lines. To get the most out of their facial cupping experience, beginners should practice gentle and consistent cupping techniques.

HANDLING PAIN DURING CUPPING

While facial cupping is generally painless, beginners may experience mild discomfort or tightness, especially if using stronger suction levels or larger cups. To minimize discomfort, start with smaller cups and gradually increase suction as your skin becomes accustomed to the sensation. Managing discomfort during facial cupping is crucial for beginners to ensure a positive and enjoyable experience.

To minimize any uncomfortable pulling or tugging sensations, it is recommended that beginners avoid sensitive areas like the eyelids and lips and concentrate instead on larger facial areas like the forehead and cheeks. A thin layer of facial oil or serum applied before cupping helps reduce friction and enhance the gliding movement of the cups across the skin.

To minimize discomfort during facial cupping, one should begin with smaller cups, use gentle suction, and apply lubrication to enable smooth movement of the cup. When comfort is given priority and techniques are tailored to the sensitivity of each individual's skin, novices can reap the restorative benefits of facial cupping without needless discomfort or irritation.

CHAPTER NINE
COMPREHENSIVE ANSWERS ON FACE CUPPING

HOW OFTEN SHOULD MY FACE BE CUPPED?

Regular facial cupping sessions can produce noticeable results for skin health and appearance. For newcomers, it is advised to begin with one to two sessions per week to give your skin time to adjust to the treatment and assess its effects. The length of each session varies from 5 to 10 minutes, depending on the sensitivity of your skin and the level of suction used. Repetition is necessary to achieve desired results; exceeding this amount may result in skin irritation or bruises.

If you would like, you can increase the frequency of facial cupping to three times a week as your skin gets used to it. However, keep in mind that the purpose of facial cupping is to gently and effectively promote lymphatic drainage, stimulate circulation, and enhance skin elasticity over time; overdoing it can strain delicate facial tissues.

Including facial cupping in your skincare routine can be a calming ritual that is best done in the evening after cleansing your face. This allows the benefits of cupping to work in tandem with your skin's natural healing processes while you sleep. The key to maximizing the benefits of facial cupping while maintaining the health and resilience of your skin is moderation and consistency.

WHAT CAN I ANTICIPATE FOLLOWING A SESSION?

Some people may experience mild bruising, especially if the suction intensity is high or if the skin is particularly delicate. This bruising usually resolves within a few days and can be minimized with lighter suction pressure during future sessions. Following a facial cupping session, it's normal to see temporary redness in the treated areas due to increased blood circulation.

This effect typically subsides within a few minutes to an hour, depending on your skin's sensitivity and the intensity of the treatment.

A revitalized appearance is one of the immediate benefits of facial cupping, as the stimulation of blood flow and lymphatic drainage helps to eliminate toxins and reduce puffiness. Regular cupping sessions can also help to improve elasticity, reduce the appearance of fine lines and wrinkles, and give your skin a more even tone over time.

A gentle, nourishing moisturizer or facial oil can help soothe any temporary sensitivity and lock in hydration.

With regular practice and appropriate aftercare, facial cupping can become a beneficial addition to your skincare routine, promoting overall skin health and radiance. Hydrating your skin after a session is important to replenish moisture and support its recovery process.

CAN WRINKLES BE REDUCED BY FACIAL CUPPING?

Frequent sessions can contribute to a more youthful-looking complexion by reducing the depth of wrinkles and improving overall skin texture. Cupping therapy is popular because of its ability to reduce the appearance of wrinkles and fine lines. It works by stimulating collagen production and promoting circulation, which over time helps plump the skin and improve its elasticity.

When done correctly, facial cupping can be a gentle yet effective way to address signs of aging and promote skin rejuvenation. The secret to getting noticeable results with facial cupping is consistency and proper technique. You should use the correct suction strength and glide the cups smoothly across your face to avoid causing unnecessary tension or skin irritation.

Although there can be noticeable changes in the texture and tone of your skin after facial cupping, you should always combine this treatment with a thorough skincare routine that protects your skin from UV rays, keeps you hydrated, and nourishes your skin with serums or creams rich in antioxidants. By combining facial cupping with these healthy habits, you can help your skin retain its natural resilience and look younger.

WHAT TIME OF DAY IS IDEAL FOR CUPPING?

A lot of practitioners advise incorporating cupping into your evening skincare ritual, ideally after cleansing your face. This timing allows the treatment to support your skin's nighttime repair processes, promoting better absorption of skincare products and maximizing its rejuvenating effects overnight. Several ways choosing the best time of day to perform facial cupping can maximize its benefits and fit seamlessly into your skincare routine.

Before bed, you can also use facial cupping to release tension that has built up during the day and to help you relax. This will help you sleep better and allow your skin to repair and regenerate. For people who have hectic schedules during the day, evening sessions may be more convenient as they offer a soothing way to end the day while putting skincare first.

Even though the evening is usually advised for facial cupping, the ideal time ultimately depends on your lifestyle and personal preferences. Some people find that cupping sessions in the morning are energizing, as they help to awaken and energize their complexion for the day. It's helpful to try out different times to see what suits your skin the best and fits in with your daily routine.

CAN CUPPING REDUCE THE PUFFINESS IN MY FACE?

Facial cupping is well known for its ability to minimize puffiness on the face and to create a more sculpted appearance. The mild suction of the cups encourages lymphatic drainage, which helps to eliminate extra fluid and toxins that cause puffiness. This can leave the complexion looking noticeably more toned and refreshed, especially in areas that are prone to swelling, like the cheeks and under the eyes.

Light gliding movements with the cups across your face encourage lymphatic circulation without causing undue pressure or discomfort. Regular practice can help to minimize puffiness over time, revealing smoother and more defined facial contours. Proper cupping technique is essential to effectively target facial puffiness.

By incorporating facial cupping into your skincare routine and using it regularly, you can support a more toned, radiant complexion while effectively addressing concerns related to facial puffiness. Facial cupping can reduce puffiness and also improve the absorption of skincare products by allowing active ingredients to penetrate deeper into the skin. This can amplify the benefits of your skincare routine and promote overall skin health.

CHAPTER TEN

USING FACE CUPPING IN CONJUNCTION WITH OTHER THERAPIES

COMBINING TRADITIONAL FACIALS WITH CUPPING

During a session, tiny suction cups are gently moved across the face, creating a vacuum effect that lifts the skin and underlying tissues, encouraging blood flow to the surface, bringing oxygen and nutrients that nourish the skin cells and promote a healthy glow. By combining cupping therapy with traditional facials, you can further stimulate circulation and lymphatic drainage, which helps to reduce puffiness, promote collagen production, and detoxify the skin. Overall, cupping therapy can improve skin health and rejuvenation.

Adding cupping to traditional facials helps improve skin health overall, leaving skin firmer, smoother, and more radiant.

Newcomers should begin with short sessions and gentle suction to acclimate the skin gradually. As they become more comfortable, they can explore longer sessions and varying techniques to tailor the treatment to their skincare goals. After cupping, the pores are temporarily opened, allowing serums and moisturizers to penetrate deeper into the skin for enhanced effectiveness.

CUPPING TO RELIEVE TMJ PAIN

Cupping applied to the jaw area helps relax tight muscles and improve circulation, reducing inflammation and promoting healing. During a session, cups are placed strategically along the jawline and temple area to target specific trigger points and tension areas. The gentle suction creates a pulling sensation that can release tightness and encourage relaxation in the jaw muscles. Cupping therapy is a non-invasive approach to alleviating discomfort related to the temporomandibular joint (TMJ).

TMJ disorders can cause jaw pain, clicking or popping sounds, and restricted movement, which is often caused by stress, teeth grinding, or misalignment.

Regular sessions can help maintain jaw flexibility and reduce the frequency and intensity of TMJ-related discomfort. Using cupping for TMJ relief is a complementary treatment that works well with other therapies like massage and stretching exercises. It can be incorporated into a comprehensive approach to managing TMJ symptoms, promoting overall jaw health and comfort. Beginners should work with a trained practitioner to ensure proper placement and technique, as well as to monitor progress over time.

COMBINING FACIAL EXERCISES WITH CUPPING

When combined with cupping therapy, which increases blood flow and collagen production, facial exercises can enhance the tone and elasticity of the muscles in the face, resulting in a more youthful appearance. For example, cupping improves circulation, which allows muscles to receive more oxygen and nutrients during exercises, which in turn helps to tone and firm the skin. Facial exercises involve specific movements and expressions designed to target muscles in the cheeks, forehead, and jawline.

Combining cupping with facial exercises also promotes lymphatic drainage, which helps to reduce puffiness and fluid retention. Initially, beginners can begin with basic exercises such as facial yoga or massage techniques that help to improve circulation and relax the face.

As they advance, they can use cupping to enhance the results of these exercises and achieve a more rejuvenated and sculpted appearance. Repetition of these techniques is essential for achieving noticeable results in terms of skin texture and facial muscle tone.

INCLUDING CUPPING IN PRACTICES FOR HOLISTIC HEALTH

While holistic health emphasizes the interconnectedness of the body, mind, and spirit, viewing health as a balance of these elements, cupping can support overall well-being by addressing both the physical and emotional aspects of health. Cupping therapy is in line with this philosophy by promoting circulation, reducing stress, and supporting detoxification. When combined with other holistic practices like acupuncture, meditation, or herbal medicine, cupping can enhance their therapeutic benefits.

When cupping is used in holistic health practices, the treatments are customized to each patient's needs and objectives. A holistic approach to health that promotes balance and vitality can be supported by cupping by treating both physical symptoms and emotional well-being. Practitioners can combine cupping with acupuncture to enhance energy flow (Qi) or with meditation to promote relaxation and mental clarity. Beginners exploring holistic health approaches can benefit from incorporating cupping as part of a comprehensive wellness routine.

AROMATHERAPY AND CUPPING TOGETHER

Aromatherapy, which uses essential oils derived from plants to promote physical and psychological benefits like relaxation, improved mood, and improved sleep quality, can intensify its therapeutic effects when combined with cupping therapy, which promotes circulation and detoxification.

During a session, cups are applied to specific areas of the body, creating a vacuum that draws blood to the surface and enhances the absorption of essential oils through the skin. Combining cupping with aromatherapy results in a synergistic approach to relaxation, stress relief, and overall well-being.

Combining cupping with aromatherapy enables a customized approach to health and well-being.

Various essential oils have distinct qualities (e.g., peppermint for energizing, lavender for relaxing, or eucalyptus for respiratory support) that enable practitioners to customize treatments to individual needs. Novices can begin by learning the fundamentals of aromatherapy blends and cupping techniques under the supervision of an aromatherapist or trained practitioner. This combination not only improves the sensory aspects of cupping but also encourages a more profound sense of relaxation and well-being, making it an invaluable complement to holistic health regimens.

CHAPTER ELEVEN

UPCOMING DEVELOPMENTS IN FACE CUPPING

NEW METHODOLOGIES AND INNOVATIONS

Recent years have seen a development in facial cupping techniques and innovations that increase its efficacy and accessibility for novices. Traditional Chinese medicine principles, which emphasize the balancing of qi and blood flow within the face, underpin many of these advancements. New techniques focus on refining cupping tools to be more ergonomic and versatile, catering specifically to facial contours. Another innovation is the introduction of silicone cups, which are softer and gentler on the skin, making them ideal for sensitive areas around the eyes and mouth.

In addition, new developments in cupping techniques highlight the significance of appropriate application techniques to avoid bruising or discomfort, ensuring a safe and effective experience for beginners.

As these techniques continue to evolve, facial cupping is becoming a versatile skincare tool that combines ancient wisdom with contemporary skincare needs, making it accessible and beneficial for all skin types. Combining cupping with serums or oils to enhance absorption and nourishment is one way that facial cupping incorporates modern skincare practices.

Technology has also contributed significantly to the advancement of facial cupping techniques. Suction control settings on tools enable novices to customize the intensity of the treatment based on comfort and skin sensitivity, resulting in a customized skincare routine. In general, these new developments and advancements in facial cupping serve novices who are looking for non-invasive, holistic skincare solutions that support youthful-looking skin.

DEVELOPMENTS IN FACIAL CUPPING RESEARCH

The physiological benefits and therapeutic effects of facial cupping have been further explored in recent years. Research has demonstrated that facial cupping improves circulation and lymphatic drainage, which assists in reducing puffiness and encourages detoxification. Cutting-edge research methodologies, such as imaging techniques and biochemical analyses, have clarified the mechanisms underlying these benefits, emphasizing the benefits of facial cupping in terms of its ability to stimulate collagen production and improve skin elasticity. These results offer scientific validation for the efficaciousness of facial cupping in combating signs of aging and enhancing overall skin vitality.

In addition, recent advancements in research have revealed particular facial pressure points that, when stimulated by cupping, can reduce stress and induce relaxation. This therapeutic benefit of facial cupping is especially attractive to novices who are looking for a natural way to decompress and rejuvenate. Studies have also looked into the potential benefits of combining facial cupping with other skincare treatments, like microdermabrasion or LED light therapy, to achieve optimal results. These studies highlight facial cupping as a flexible skincare modality that can be customized to address a wide range of skin concerns successfully.

Beginning with an understanding of the physiological mechanisms and therapeutic benefits validated through research, beginners can confidently incorporate facial cupping into their skincare routines, knowing they are harnessing the power of both ancient wisdom and modern scientific insights. As research in facial cupping continues to evolve, the integration of evidence-based practices into skincare routines offers beginners a scientifically supported approach to achieving healthy and radiant skin.

POPULARITY AND CELEBRITY ENDORSEMENTS

Celebrities who are looking for effective skincare solutions have been endorsing facial cupping, which has helped it become more popular among those starting.

Celebrities have been praising facial cupping for its ability to improve facial contours, reduce puffiness, and impart a glowing complexion. Their endorsements on social media platforms and red carpets, along with their testimonials, have sparked curiosity and interest in facial cupping as a non-invasive alternative to surgical procedures.

Celebrity skincare routines frequently include facial cupping as a crucial step in achieving camera-ready skin, emphasizing its effectiveness in delivering visible results quickly. Additionally, the endorsement of skincare experts and influencers has further cemented facial cupping's status as a mainstream skincare practice. These endorsements highlight the versatility of facial cupping in addressing various skin concerns, from fine lines to uneven skin tone, making it a versatile tool in the pursuit of youthful and radiant skin.

With tutorials and guidance from influencers and skincare professionals, beginners can learn proper techniques and application methods to maximize the benefits of facial cupping. As celebrity endorsements continue to drive interest in facial cupping, its popularity among beginners seeking effective and natural skincare solutions is expected to grow. The availability of facial cupping tools endorsed by celebrities has made it easier for beginners to incorporate this practice into their daily skincare routines at home.

ECO-FRIENDLINESS IN CUPPING TECHNIQUES

Sustainable cupping practices emphasize the use of eco-friendly materials for cupping tools, such as silicone or recyclable materials, reducing environmental impact. Manufacturers are increasingly adopting sustainable production methods that minimize waste and carbon footprint, ensuring that facial cupping remains a responsible choice for beginners and skincare enthusiasts alike. The integration of sustainable practices into facial cupping is in line with the growing global awareness of environmental conservation and ethical consumption.

In addition, ethical sourcing of ingredients for skincare products that are used in conjunction with cupping treatments is another aspect of sustainable cupping practices. Organic and cruelty-free skincare formulations are a great complement to facial cupping, promoting holistic skincare routines that prioritize skin health and environmental stewardship. Even beginners can embrace sustainable cupping practices with confidence, knowing that their skincare choices have a positive impact on both environmental sustainability and ethical standards.

WORKSHOPS AND EDUCATIONAL MATERIALS

Online platforms offer virtual workshops that provide step-by-step guidance on facial cupping techniques, ensuring beginners understand the principles and benefits before practicing at home. These workshops often include demonstrations and Q&A sessions to address common concerns and ensure beginners feel confident in their skincare routines. The availability of educational resources and workshops has democratized access to knowledge about facial cupping, empowering beginners to learn proper techniques and application methods from certified professionals.

Expert-led tutorials emphasize safety protocols and hygiene practices to prevent adverse reactions and maximize the benefits of facial cupping. Beginners can access comprehensive guides and instructional videos that break down each step of facial cupping, from preparation to post-treatment care, fostering a supportive learning environment. Educational resources also offer in-depth insights into the history and cultural significance of facial cupping, connecting novices with its rich traditions in holistic wellness.

Education and workshops help beginners become proficient in facial cupping techniques and effectively integrate them into their skincare rituals for long-term skin health and rejuvenation.

The abundance of online educational resources also encourages beginners to experiment with different variations of facial cupping, such as lymphatic drainage techniques or acupressure points tailored to individual skin concerns. Advanced workshops delve into advanced topics, such as integrating facial cupping with skincare modalities like gua sha or microcurrent therapy, expanding beginners' knowledge and skill set.

www.ingramcontent.com/pod-product-compliance
Lightning Source LLC
Chambersburg PA
CBHW061252250726
48653CB00002B/623

9798333682024